NO MEDALS FOR M.E.

LISETTE SKEET

Strategic Book Publishing and Rights Co.

Strategic Book Publishing and Rights Co., LLC
USA | Singapore
www.sbpra.com

For information about special discounts for bulk purchases, please contact Strategic Book Publishing and Rights Co., LLC Special Sales, at bookorder@sbpra.net.

ISBN: 978-1-68181-497-1

For Your Future Well Self

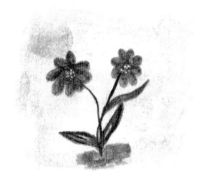

CONTENTS

INTRODUCTION

I wanted to write this book some years ago. In diaries, I recorded what happened to me, with all the difficulties I faced and the enormous effort I made to recover. I knew I would never forget how wonderful it felt to be well at last and longed to help others who were diagnosed with the same condition. Often, in conversation, no matter how enthusiastic I was, I found people seemed to be contemptuous of my experience, even disbelieving, so that, every time I tried to explain what I did and the results I experienced, I would be beaten back — especially by those who never had it themselves!

I have found it hard to bear stories in the media about victims of myalgic encephalomyelitis who suffer for years with no hope of regaining strength and wellbeing. I feel concerned when post-viral fatigue is mixed up with the awful M.E., even though some symptoms do cross-over.

Over twenty years ago, I decided I had to put the many months of illness behind me as best I could. Being doubted hurt. I hoped someone else would be able to describe, in a useful way, the type of recovery I made. As there have been times when I learned of individuals who actually gave up on life completely, hid from daylight or even died, it has been very difficult to keep away from the debate. After all that time, I suddenly realised something:

"Okay ... so I am not a doctor ... but I am honest and I *can tell*

1

you what happened to me!"

My experience was a long time ago but I am the same person, albeit older and sometimes I return to my own way of gaining the best chance of good health, in order to recover from a viral illness or a phase of feeling exhausted. I still have weak arms and a familiar ache when I try to reach up for any length of time but otherwise I am able to enjoy being well, even though I live with the memories of how I got better from my illness and what a gift the renewal of good health was.

My Baby

During the spring of 1987, at the age of thirty-two, I was very well and felt strong, confident and peaceful in myself. I had a lively six-year-old son and expected a second child in May. When I went to a neighbour's make-up party the demonstrator lightly touched the tanned and freckled skin on my face with her forefinger, saying: "Your skin is *lovely and normal* across there, isn't it?"

At last my due date was close and I pottered about in my bedroom, folding tiny clothes and preparing items to take with me for labour. As I carried a case to the uncarpeted wooden staircase in our old cottage, I was careless and probably moving too fast considering how big my bump had grown. I missed a step and slipped, from about halfway down the stairs to the foot. However, getting up quickly I felt unhurt. My husband installed me in an armchair and made tea, after which we might have forgotten my tumble but during the night contractions began, becoming increasingly relentless so that, by the early hours of the next day, I needed to go to the maternity ward of the nearby hospital.

It was to be a long time afterwards, when I reflected upon how I came to be treated casually by midwives, that I realised the trigger for labour must have been that fall and the process might not have happened for a day or two otherwise.

Nurses were insistent that I was mistaken in identifying contractions. I should not have arrived there yet, they said and added, to my horror, that I was to go home! I could not believe it. I had coped quietly for several hours but I needed professional support at that point, since I was having regular pains, using breathing exercises in order to withstand them. For sure, I had begun early stages of giving birth but they flatly refused to give me a private space and I was forced to leave, with every fibre of my being resisting the act of standing to walk, let alone travel all the way back to the cottage and imagine nothing was happening! Argument was hopeless and I felt afraid.

I could barely make it back to the car. As my husband drove, I tried to relax through contractions but it was almost impossible with a racing heart and we both struggled to comprehend that I had to turn away from the hospital.

That afternoon, my doctor was called and he arrived at the cottage quickly, even though it was a Sunday. He did not need to examine me, before he made an urgent telephone call to staff in the maternity ward and I could tell he was trying to control incredulity and some anger. Upon his insistence, we went back and although I was terribly uncomfortable during the drive I was very glad to be heading in the right direction! Soon, I began to receive the essential nursing care I deserved.

"Well," commented a midwife, not unkindly, "*you* don't do things in the usual way, do you?" My body plunged into the pushing stage and my second son was born safely at seven o'clock that evening, May twenty-fourth, 1987. Late sunshine shone through the window, touching his small head and turning the soft fuzz of dark hair to a shade of golden-brown.

Unfortunately, I was in physical and mental distress as a result of the forced travelling whilst I was vulnerable and although it was essentially a normal birth, I was dreadfully tired. That night the baby was restless, having been affected by an inevitably belated dose of pethidine and I was unable to sleep.

The Start

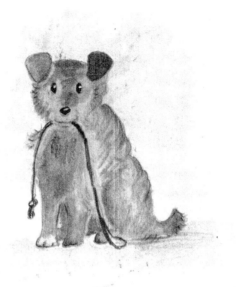

I was thrilled with my new baby and looked forward to taking him home to meet his brother; as we both seemed well, we left the hospital the next day. Within the same week however, I knew something was wrong with me since I felt odd and kept breaking into hot sweats, also I was constantly nauseous. I took little notice of all this and could not have guessed what was to come.

All summer, I fought maddening physical weakness to carry on caring for my children. One day my older son wanted to go to a local fete. It was not far away but the task of preparing to go and then the short walk there seemed enormous. I felt better as I sat in the sun but I was soon to be much worse.

By the autumn I was becoming really ill with a number of confusing symptoms; these included repeated bouts of cystitis as well as a persistent sore throat. I got a cold, then another that felt so bad I thought it must be the flu' since I ached all over and my face burned. If anyone asked me how I was, I would sing the praises of my baby but add honestly that I seemed to keep getting a viral illness, saying, "I'm *so* fed up — I can't seem to shake it off!"

A Doctor

Days grew shorter and the weather turned cold. One afternoon, I lay on my bed in a state of despair, absolutely floored by weakness and exhaustion and the way my head relentlessly ached. I had tried very hard to be active for days before this but now I was forced to admit that I was very unwell indeed. A young doctor came to see me (they would, in those days!); he was not the one who knew me and almost as soon as he walked into the room, it felt impossible to get his full attention. Normally eloquent, I could not think how to express myself and no matter how carefully I described my collapse, symptoms did not sound serious and there was no way to emphasise my distress. (It did not occur to me to throw a tantrum but I was not strong enough to do that anyway!) The doctor was impatient; he fidgeted about and avoided looking at me. Instead, he stood at the foot of the bed, where, asking if this was a listed building, he interested himself in the oak beams of our cottage!

I had such a sense of disappointment and frustration, (it was to become a familiar feeling) and in addition, I was scared — what on earth was happening? When the doctor left he had not examined me or offered anything useful, except to say my condition would doubtless improve.

BETTER?

On I went, sometimes feverish, having daily headaches and always feeling very tired. I would fall asleep whilst the baby napped and go to bed at night as early as I could. It is so easy for others to dismiss the ailments of a new mother as being part of the busy and sometimes stressful side of caring for young children but at Christmas my mother-in-law agreed to look after my older son and I had a very peaceful day, quietly caring for the baby, tidying around the house, not analysing what had been happening to me. I made a meal for myself and my husband, thinking simply:

"Hooray! I feel better!"

I really did. Symptoms went away, I was young and happy (no time in my life has ever been nicer than when I had a new baby to care for; I know I was lucky not to suffer from post-natal depression); with no reason to fear my illness would return I was only too glad to put it all behind me.

In January, feeling sure I was quite well and not a bit concerned to worry further about the difficulties I had been through, I decided to treat myself to a horse ride. Why would I expect renewed problems? I had enjoyed good health, in the past!

I loved being at the stables and leaned my cheek against the warm dun-coloured neck of a friendly cob as I tightened the girth and fastened stirrup leathers. The stocky little horse was an unbalanced and bumpy mount; almost as soon as we set off, I became aware that I was in trouble. Despite being competent on horseback I lost my posture, breathing heavily. As the leader of the ride encouraged us to follow at a trot, enthusiastically keeping up a fast pace, I felt the old sensation of a falling-away of my strength. I kept quiet and got to the end of the hour somehow but I had really done the trick — now I was ill again.

At home, I collapsed into fatigue, nausea, headaches, pain and the rest.

Sunday Lunch

Days passed and although I powerfully resisted the emotional and physical effects of illness, I was almost unable to cope. Caring for the boys went to the top of the list, then the pets (a little dog and a cat). I had times when I could not add much in the way of personal care to the list of things I absolutely had to get done.

One Sunday I was persuaded to go out for lunch with some friends. It is natural for those around a chronically sick person to offer ideas for feeling better and I went along with the notion that a change of scene and a special meal might help, even though, in my heart, I knew I was not up to it, especially when my companions wanted to sit in a pub garden. It would have certainly made me feel good if an outing was the right decision but although it was not a cold day I felt deeply chilled and with my head and shoulders wrapped in a thick scarf, I was informed, too jovially, that I looked like "an old woman".

I had little appetite but drank some wine; however it made me feel worse instead of better and later, at home, I felt hellish. I wondered if there was anything I could take to relieve my misery and wandered into the bathroom, where I stared pointlessly at a medicine cabinet.

The Symptoms

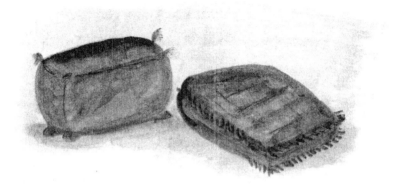

These are the symptoms I suffered and sometimes there were an awful lot of them, all at once:

Headaches, often appalling in intensity. Dizziness. Poor concentration. Poor eyesight. Tiredness and sleepiness. Chest pain and coughing. Very sore throat. Cystitis. Weak muscles and poor grip in the hands. Irregular periods. A sense of deep sorrow. Profound emotional sensitivity to serious or frightening news items. Feeling cold or sometimes, far too hot, with facial flushing. Pain in the long muscles of my arms and legs.

I believe my whole system was completely upset by the experience at the maternity ward. At a crucial time when I needed responsible, professional assistance, I was turned away and could not avoid feeling deeply unnerved — so I suffered shock and fear *in addition to* the usual trials of labour. As a direct result of being treated with casual contempt, physically and emotionally I was overwhelmed.

THE REAL ME

In my life before those days, I never felt depressed. I was active, an animal lover and an able rider, an energetic swimmer; in addition, I was fiercely independent and very proud of my little family. The reactions of other people when I could not pretend to be in good health, began to be a serious worry; I felt baffled. It was painful to realise, gradually, with a sense of shock every time this was highlighted, that I was perceived as being fussy and lazy by now! It seemed unnatural — surely I might have expected to be at least *partly* understood?

By the time my littlest boy neared his first birthday, I was in a bad way. For reasons I am not going to examine in depth in terms of the psychology behind them, almost no-one was interested in helping me when some gestures of kindly support would have eased my suffering and my soul.

I read in the newspaper that a type of illness called "Yuppie Flu" had been identified! Not only did it bear a silly name, it was described derisively as if sufferers *wanted* to be unwell, yet symptoms resembled my condition and they were anything but funny.

One afternoon, I went slowly across the village green at the front of the cottage to meet my older son as he returned from primary school. I wore two coats to protect me from shivering as soon as I was out in the fresh air and at a much later date, I was to learn neighbours were gossiping, saying I had put on weight! As I stood near another mother, we chatted. It might have been nice for by then I was often lonely; sometimes I could barely speak. However, when I mentioned what I read and was thinking about myself, she said, rudely:

"Hah, just because you saw something in a paper, doesn't mean you have it!" I gave up on an explanation, wondering nevertheless why I may not identify my illness.

THE DIAGNOSIS

It was nightmarish to go on feeling ill; I *had* to be enabled to move on! Before long, I returned to the surgery where I managed to persuade my family doctor I had a set of symptoms that did not make sense. After describing concerns upon reading and recognising descriptions of the supposed phenomenon called Yuppie Flu; at last, I was referred to a specialist and a letter to confirm the appointment duly arrived. This time I was properly examined. Sitting with my legs crossed, I had a test, the simple tap on part of the knee for reflexes: I had none! This mightily satisfied the consultant since it was, apparently *classic*! I was an M.E. sufferer.

I waited … Here was, I knew, an important diagnosis from which I hoped with all my heart to go forward, better-equipped to make a full recovery. Nothing was forthcoming! Seated on that chair in a chilly room, incredulously, I received the information that "some people get better…."

So, I wanted to know, how long would the illness last? The doctor could not say and that was all that happened; the consultation had lasted just a few minutes.

I was not asked, by this person who had a "special interest" in M.E. (yet no interest in me it seemed), about how I feel and act when I am well; what I thought might have precipitated my collapse or how I was managing the condition. No comments were made about medicines, nutrition or pain management and there was nothing useful of any description, to take away with me. Was I part of an experiment, sent home with absolutely no form of support *to see what would happen?*

That evening, a kind aunt who was beginning to be concerned for me after hearing something of my troubles, called on the telephone. She was the only person who showed any interest in how I got on. She felt frustrated as she lived too far away to help but asked, was it better to know for sure that I had a label for the condition? I hardly knew. Was it? What had I gained, in reality?

After the hospital visit, as others gradually caught up with the information I had been given, many adopted an air of annoyance that seemed strange … were they *cross* with me? I could not bear it; for days, there were tears at the back of my eyes and tightness in my throat as I struggled to believe that the sensible and cheerful character I had been in the past, now counted for nothing. Even with a diagnosis, I was suspected of malingering!

Tears

I learned, eventually, not to cry about having *myalgic encephalomy-elitis*. I stood in the kitchen one day and looked around the room at all the things waiting to be done ... I wanted to get on with cleaning counters and the refrigerator, collecting up toys and caring properly for our pets. In frustration *then*, I broke down but when the bout of tears passed, sadly, I thought:

"No-one knows when I'm crying. It wastes my strength — I might as well not do it because it's completely pointless!" After that, I very rarely wept; I knew that I was in this fix on my own.

During one of her rare visits, my mother seemed dismissive of my diagnosis and cross that I could not go for a walk. She described my younger sister, who was apparently looking "really fresh, in her blue jeans and a white shirt, with her hair all shiny!" My sister had every right to be on top form but I found a tiny reserve of spirit:

"You know — either of my sisters could get this illness." Her beautiful sapphire-blue eyes glanced briefly at me but then flickered away and she answered:

"*They* wouldn't ...!"

How *did* she contemplate my wan and ailing figure and fail to care? At the window, as my small son stood on a stool and waved, I watched her walk away, upright and smart in a new coat, not, apparently, wondering how I would cope for the rest of that day and in those to come.

I found a stack of old magazines and looked for an "agony aunt". Several women appeared to fit the description in those days but I chose one who was thought to have gravitas, since she was a trained nurse and battled a long-term physical problem of her own which made her compassionate — or so one thought. Feeling desperate, I managed to write to her and explained frankly:

"This is not the real "me"! I am nearly mad from weakness and inability to do what I want!" I made it as clear as I could and insisted I was usually energetic and confident. I had to write my appeal in two parts but once it was ready my young son took it to the letterbox nearby on the village green, then I waited ... and I *really hoped* for a good outcome.

* * *

A letter came in response and it was a personal reply, the envelope was handwritten and two typed sheets inside were signed but I stared in disbelief at the words, which included a disingenuous suggestion that I look for a reason for the way I felt. Had I tried exercise? It was the same hurtful rubbish I read in newspapers. Presumptive and patronising, the lady said *she did not believe M.E. is a real illness.*

NANA

My maternal grandmother, who had not, so far, responded to the few snippets of information from the rest of the family, had something of a change of heart after my condition was diagnosed. As an extraordinarily lively eighty-year-old, she often complained of boredom in her tiny house in the north of the country. Nana loved looking after people, especially children, so it was wonderful when she came to stay with us and bravely took on the challenge of managing the household, for a time. She cooked, cleaned, took my older son to school and trundled the little one out for rides in his pushchair, each afternoon. During their "breathers" as Nana termed these trips around the village, feeling comforted because I had support and could lean, just a bit, on another, I fell helplessly asleep!

One day, Nana weighed herself on our bathroom scales. She came to stand before me; a small figure in the setting of our cottage living-room making a picture which my memory recorded in photographic perfection. She was immaculate, with short hair, smart sandals on her feet, a brown wool dress with a neat collar and a narrow gold belt around her trim waist.

"What do you think I weigh?" she demanded. The answer popped into my head and I knew!

"Eight-and-a-half stones?"

"*Exactly*!" She beamed, nodded and trotted off very contentedly, whilst I lay back on the settee. I was the poor soul at the age of thirty-three! At eighty, my grandmother was fine!

Nana's wellness must have been partly good luck, since she certainly had her share of tragedy and hard times. However, she ate a sensible diet, including plenty of fruit and vegetables. She disliked most types of alcohol, although she would allow herself a minute glass of sweet sherry, to be festive at Christmas-time. Like me, she did not smoke. She was a person who naturally sought out healthy foods; in addition, she loved to be out in the fresh air, preferably by the sea.

As for me, I was not in a condition that would cheer anyone's heart and had not realised I could try a nutritional approach. I was pathetic in the true sense of the word, in my weak inability to express myself or move freely, still terribly confused about what was happening to me and worrying about why I had to suffer. Nana tired of all this eventually and returned to her home.

TIME

Time passed and my gait became jerky when I walked. My world narrowed and I rarely saw a change of scene; had I been offered an outing in a wheelchair I would have been deeply grateful. Before long, since I was forced to put my scant energies into caring for the boys, I had nothing left for myself. I could not wash my hair or peg washing on a line; if I dropped a tissue I could hardly bend to pick it up. Occasionally the telephone rang and I had to ignore it, with no voice to talk and a growing fear of being hurt by careless comment since the honest answer to even a casual query had to be: "I feel very ill".

In an ideal marriage, my husband would have been fully able to support and comfort me but he really did not understand what was happening, any more than I did. He worked longer and longer hours and at a later date it was revealed he had been struggling to save his business as an economic recession approached.

My hopes of feeling better were fading and it was a painful process, especially as I was living in a pretty cottage in a Suffolk village, loved being a mother and life could have been good. A neighbour, when she learned that I was an experienced rider, asked me to exercise her mare, kindly saying I was welcome to ride at any time. How frustrating — *if only I could!*

I went to bed at night with a prayer that I would awaken next day feeling better but I slept on the nasty feeling that I would not.

It was disastrous. I became cross and sad; losing sight of the real "me" I thought: *"No good can come of this!"*

M.E. victims know only too well that a psychoanalyst might at this point comment: "You knew you would not feel better? That's why you didn't!" Uh huh? **No.**

One afternoon, feeling sick and shaky, I supplied my toddler with crayons and paper and he sat contentedly on the bed, scribbling and chatting while I dozed. I heard the door open downstairs and felt a tiny hope as a voice called my name. It was a friend … well, sort of. She peered into the bedroom briefly and said she had come to collect some kitchen equipment, lent some months before. As I forced away my pride, the question had to be asked:

"Have you time to help me?"

Falsely jovial, she replied, "not today!" Did she think a cheerful disregard for my suffering meant it could be chased away? She did. "I'm baking for charity!"

Other people went away on holidays, enjoyed sports or careers … They could get on with their lives but I had to crawl through my days. I hung on somehow to dreams of recovery, yet I had no idea how to make them come true and began to succumb to a sense of hopelessness. I could not explain my plight when all I encountered was refusal to listen.

A PARCEL

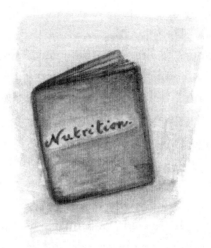

One person seemed to take on board the reality of my situation. An aunt, the kind lady who called to ask about the diagnosis, clearly believed me and she mentioned the M.E. Association. Remembering, I managed to trace the telephone number, made a brief call and was sent pamphlets, which I read a little at a time as the text seemed to jump about before my eyes. The piece of information about potential recovery, which had seemed so weak coming from the consultant, suddenly took on a new importance: ***Some people recover.***

So .... I was highly unlikely to die of my illness and I did not want to remain debilitated. If it was true that some sufferers recover — I wanted to be in that number!

On a chilly day in early spring, when my older son was in school, his little brother was very lively. He would be two years old in a couple of months. I got him into a jacket and he pulled on his boots then ran to the back door but I could not risk opening it until I was ready.

"Can you find your scarf?" I suggested and he cheerfully trotted off to his room, whilst I laboriously put on layers of warm clothing and wrapped my head and shoulders in a thick blanket. Now we could go outside although I shuffled just a few paces to the picnic table, where I sat and watched as my child busily dug in a pile of sand with a plastic spade; I hoped he would not make a dash for the gateway!

My boys were the focus of my life and there were so many things I wanted to do with them. I remembered a tale I read in articles about the so-called Yuppie Flu, a year before. Perhaps it was an urban myth. An M.E. victim was thrown into a swimming pool, to call his bluff and see if he would swim ... of course, somehow, he did stay afloat and this was supposed to prove he was not ill in the first place. It sounded so cruel, I always hoped it was untrue. If my son ran off I knew I would force myself to catch him but it did not change the fact that I was ill and weak.

As I sat there, I knew a sense of despair and since I was almost positive that I would never be well; there seemed to be nothing to look forward to. A blackbird sang and feeling disorientated I looked up at the branches of an apple tree where it perched, as I heard the sound of footsteps crunching on the gravel in the driveway and the postman made his over way to me . No doubt this was an ordinary day for him. For me, as he handed over a parcel wrapped in brown paper, secured with sticky tape and covered in labels, it was about to become wonderful.

When I recognised my aunt's curly handwriting I smiled. Words cannot fully describe how thrilled I felt to receive a present! I was *so* lonely, even if there had been something dull inside, I would have felt just a tiny bit better.

However, there were good things to unpack — books, some new, some obviously well-read. They were all on the subject of nutrition, the best foods to eat, the vitamins and the results of deficiency in the human diet. There was one about how to manage terrible headaches; another contained descriptions of how human beings evolved and what modern eating habits might be doing to our systems.

I tucked the precious bundle into my lap and sat on, watching my son play. I had been struggling for some time to read at all but I determined to examine these books. I would begin to learn from them — *at last, I had something to go on!*

A Willing Suspension
of Disbelief

My resolve to recover returned and I began to read, sometimes just a page at a time. I researched and made my plans, although since I was weakened by long months of illness, my faith was as fragile as my health and I wavered often. When I was able to walk, I would wander along the grassy space in front of our cottage, where there were swings and children played. I would stop and lean on a stick a few times as I slowly crossed the apparently vast distance to a seat nearby … but it is not far, in reality.

"Diet cannot tackle this monster", I thought, contemplating disappointment. Yet, I had nothing else to try, there was no medication offered to me and I needed to hang on to my hopes.

My body needed a high level of meticulous care; at last I was learning that and truly, I was on the right track!

Everyone Feels Tired

My mother was a creative person who drew and painted, sewed, decorated, gardened and made her home lovely in very many ways. Naturally beautiful and immensely energetic, she did not understand my illness or respect my struggle with its effects; emphatically, she refused to involve herself in my situation.

At a time of extreme debilitation, I knew my parents were planning a dinner party. Beautiful crockery and cutlery were arrayed on a festive table, flowers decorated the room and hot food was ready. It was, of course, their business but it was a painful fact that I was not invited and nobody was coming to help me. I heard they told friends that I was "just depressed" and it was some time before I reflected that this was doubly insulting! They could not accept I had M.E. but if I *had* been depressed (a nasty condition in itself), it seemed they would have been contemptuous.

Before Nana went back to her home in the north of the country, I guessed she must have discussed my situation with my mother, who visited me once or twice during the following month and brought a basket of groceries each time. One day, she switched on the oven, put a piece of fresh chicken inside and said on leaving:

"You will get the veg', won't you?" It was not a question really and I expect she thought she was making me do something I must try. I was helpless and afraid to argue so I struggled to lift the baking tray from the oven and the little boys and I ate the baked meat with bread and tomatoes. It was all I could do.

On a morning when I was almost without resources my husband had gone away, as he often did and I sat by the telephone, wrestling with my pride before calling my parents. My father answered. He had been silent, making no observation up until now, on my condition.

"Could someone help me today?" I asked. "I am very weak …" He said: "Lis', *everyone feels tired* sometimes." Incredulous, I put the receiver down; I really was alone with my illness and my wobbly plans.

In years to come, I kept up a semblance of normality with my family. I never stopped loving my parents, who adored their grandchildren and often arranged very happy times for them. When each one passed away (my mother tragically young) I grieved deeply over their loss of life. However, I know for sure that I would never turn my back on a child of my own, no matter how grown-up the son or daughter, or how confused I might be about the reasons for any collapse.

This is not a deeply analytical story; I have studied psychoanalysis and love the process (although it can be painful) but I am leaving most of that aside for the purposes of describing my experience of illness and recovery.

NUTRITION, REST AND RECOVERY

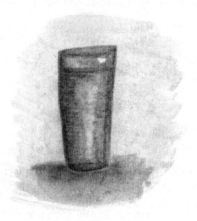

Water: This is simple: We all need to keep ourselves hydrated. As a rule, I rarely drank water but it was easy to alter this and I began to keep a glassful on the kitchen window-sill, another in the sitting room and one on a table beside my bed. I did not drink too much (apparently, one can!) but I made sure I had enough.

Putting foods right: I began to change my intake, so that I included fresh fruit and vegetables, lean meat and fish, wholemeal bread and flour … well, we know don't we? Magazines, books and news items about nutrition abound nowadays whereas in the 1980's, they were not as common. My point is this:

Instead of convincing myself that I already ate well, I took a long, hard look at my usual diet and *found it wanting*.

Vitamins and Supplements: This could be a big part of a book like mine. However, especially with access to the Internet, it is not hard to research the vitamins and what they do for us along with the way a human being may suffer if the body is depleted of the right spectrum. I opened my mind on this. It was not a time to imagine I knew better than the optimum recommendations —

clearly, I did not, since I was so ill. Planning, I decided (of course with a care for what an overdose might do) to add in some extras that might help. Simply then, I added, daily: a multivitamin pill, folic acid and a cod liver oil capsule. *I am just telling you. That is what I did.*

Sugar and Caffeine: The following is what I believe: The M.E. sufferer is extremely sensitive. A healthy person can enjoy a little sugar hit or a boost from some tea or coffee and feel nothing detrimental afterwards but I needed to achieve a comfortable plateau. That is, if sugar or caffeine sent me UP (even a little), the inevitable "coming down" could be too tiring whilst I was already weak. I sacrificed the *ups* to stop the *downs* and sought a happy medium. It is tenuous but it was pointless to dismiss the idea while I needed to make all the efforts I possibly could. This was an approach that formed a part of the whole plan and it worked for me. (See my Collapsed Puppet theory.)

Taking out the "bad": I swapped shop-bought cakes for buttered brown toast and as I grew stronger, I cooked for myself and made buns with wholemeal flour and honey to sweeten. I ate comforting foods like jacket potatoes filled with grated cheese or coleslaw. Instead of ordinary tea or coffee, I drank herbal teas, peppermint or camomile (there are lots to choose from). At first, they tasted odd but I came to like them and therefore did not feel deprived of a comforting hot drink. For breakfast, instead of sweet cereal I would have warm porridge with a spoonful of cream and a few sultanas; or a boiled egg and toast or a crumpet. I drank a glassful of freshly-squeezed orange juice, so the Vitamin C ensured absorption of iron from the egg. During the long months of illness, I had become thin, so I made cheese pastas or salad sandwiches instead of sweet things and never let myself feel wobbly from hunger. Sardines-on-toast were one of my favourite teatime meals (the fish is good for the brain). I learned to seek out fruits to satisfy sweet cravings and tried some I had neglected before, such as kiwi, pears and mango.

Variety: I achieved the best results if I avoided repetitive eating, so I tried to be imaginative and not rely on just a small selection of foods.

At first as I studied and planned a recovery, there was no option to taking as much rest as possible and I fell asleep as often as I could allow myself to do so, when the boys were in bed or if my older son was in school and little one napped. I would doze by his side, holding a piece of his jumper whilst he played with toys. They were both, thankfully, peaceable souls!

I learned from the horse-riding episode not to force myself to be active. During the long months of confusion before my diagnosis, I did what I could all the time, pushing myself to work hard but of course, I was the worse for it.

As I grew increasingly well, the need to sleep eased and I became stronger. Days suddenly seemed to hold more hours than they had for many months! Hope grew, as I examined what all the various vitamins and minerals in a good diet can offer. I looked at the ailments which research has proven arise from deficiency and learned to discard the old, obvious thoughts, such as: "How can I be deficient, when I eat all sorts of foods?"

Instead, I considered new possibilities and tried to care about myself enough to relax. Perhaps, so ill, I really did need times of peaceful sleep when the rest of the world was busy? I had stopped punishing myself. I was getting there.

I am not going to reference any of the books I read. Sometimes during my study, I would come across a proposal I did not agree with or tried and found to be problematic and in any case, I know that, supplied with a list of my favourite books, some "expert" would turn out to know for sure that approaches I adopted have been discredited … *even though I recovered.*

I am not medically-trained but awareness developed, especially when my efforts worked, that I have an analytical and in some respects, a scientific mind. In practice, I simply selected and tried —

as wisely as I could — all the approaches to good health via nutrition that I saw as potentially useful.

Note that I did not have: diabetes, asthma, arthritis or other health issues. That is, I clearly did not have to be careful about how my plan affected me **except for my M.E.**

My Body is not my Enemy!

Of course, I was tempted, in a natural response, to hate all the symptoms I suffered and yet I think they were my body's way of yelling for help. My whole system was going wrong, off-balance after the terrible shock, frustration and physical trauma I suffered whilst in a vulnerable state, at the maternity hospital. Ailments were showing me where I needed to take care.

On a serious note, during the few early days of withdrawal from a food or drink I had been having regularly, there was a sense of deep exhaustion and some nasty headaches. When this happened, holding on to hope, I ploughed on. I got rid of sugar and caffeine (one at a time) from my diet and my diaries looked something like this:

Day 1 "Quite shaky, ate a lot of fruit!"
Day 2 "Headache kicked in and was awful by teatime. It's making me miserable."
Day 3 "Still got a headache, feeling horrible and very sleepy; I keep having weird dreams."
Day 4 "Pain has gone! I'm feeling much better!"

I was absolutely prepared to feel rough for a few days to earn the reward of a true recovery, so I rested as much as I could, took painkillers and longed for the process to be over. After about four days, often it was. Sometimes I would feel disappointed if I lapsed again into headaches but since I kept on with my nutritious diet and determined exclusion of sugars and caffeine, disappointments tended to be short-lived, with a significant improvement afterwards.

My diary was also full of descriptions of how I felt, with notes on emotional ups and downs, all my efforts and the results. Such a record can become obsessional but it was a useful way to consider how I was getting on, especially as no-one would listen. However, it was absolutely no use as proof of my plan at a later date and disbelievers simply insist I fooled myself! I was certainly self-absorbed but I had to be; my target was to get myself well ... did anyone else have a better idea? No, so I had no choice.

DIFFICULTIES

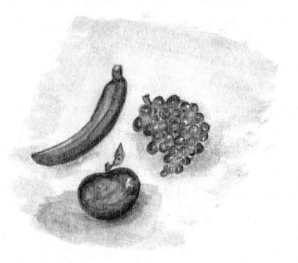

There are those who must challenge a self-help approach to fitness. Sometimes it is in the form of a careless comment, such as a response to your efforts to manage exhaustion with: "Oh, everyone gets that sometimes!" or (if you dare describe your diet!) "Food doesn't make you ill, look at me! I eat junk all the time and I am fine!" Lucky that-person then. He or she does not have M.E. and has no need to comprehend how utterly desperate I was and how I reached out for my glimmer of hope.

It is a genuine shame that the sufferer often feels unable to fully describe all the symptoms. Wouldn't it be nice if he or she had the luxury of getting bored with the whole thing? When I developed a habit of writing everything in my diary it got the agony out in a way that did not, apparently, get on someone's nerves. A word of caution: In those days we had no Facebook and I did not own a computer. Nowadays, many problems are aired in chat sites but personally I would avoid doing that so that I could work independently, without losing confidence in an argument.

More upsetting for me, was when, with no actual experience to better-inform their remarks, people apparently took an interest in my story then hit me with a rude response. A health visitor listened to my expressions of relief, when I was newly-recovered. Similar in her reaction to the agony aunt, to whom I once wrote a hopeful appeal for help, she said: "I must take issue with you! I'm not convinced you had M.E."

"Must you?" I thought. "Take *issue with me*? After everything I .... ?" I stayed silent because I had to protect my emotions but I never forgot how painful it was to be doubted!

During the same period of recent recovery, someone who knew me well even said she reckoned she had more lines on her face than me because she had seen "hard times"! I was bemused. I do not know why I stayed line-free (unless it is another great effect of a healthy diet) but most definitely I suffered hard times!

Surely, people who argued against the reality of the illness, my experiences and my mind-set; those who patronised me or showed open contempt must have felt challenged. What needs did I have that they could not be asked to meet and how unwelcome were the thoughts that arose?

HELP

I began to be very positive, albeit still physically weak; I had a plan and perhaps it shone through my feeble actions. Bizarrely, the better I seemed in every way, the oftener I saw a more compassionate response from family and friends and at last, a lady was employed, to help in my home.

This kind soul would bustle in, fill the kettle, wash a sink full of dirty crockery, load the washing machine then hang clothes on the line, sweep up, mop floors and energetically polish furniture. She chatted kindly to my little boys; I could even leave them in her care for a while and go to bed, which blessed relief really cheered and helped me. When I came downstairs to see her off, everything would be spotlessly clean with a scent of lavender in the air. The good-natured support offered by this lady, who never once said or seemed to harbour any word of hurtful or malicious comment, lifted my spirits and strengthened my resolve.

Along with my determination to care for my children, I had simpler wishes. I wanted to go to the shops in town and choose my own magazine! To browse the health food shops instead of weakly having to beg someone to bring herbal teas, seed loaves and honey. I longed to choose birthday gifts, treats from the beauty counters and I planned to hunt for interesting toys for my toddler. I could hardly envisage a day when I would be fit enough to risk it, in terms of the action and the sugar hit — but I wanted to choose my own cream cake!

One day when my housekeeper arrived, I had already cleared the washing-up! I had a straight back and better use of my arms; I was very proud. I took my patient little terrier out for a walk in the sun, it was wonderful, after all that time … I could get the lead … leave the house *and walk!* I was free from physical pain and there was relief in my heart, potentially joy.

Something was not better though and that was the hurt; it haunted me. I passed allotments and when I saw an elderly gentleman stooping over his rake I was reminded of my father and his comment, "everyone feels tired". As the thought crossed my mind, I actually heard myself sob, in an involuntary cry of sorrow.

GOING ON

Subtle changes in responses from family and friends went on. I got a few visitors. My mother came, with presents and sweets for the children, who were now aged eight and two. She told me a close friend had called her in a distressed state to say her own daughter had been given a diagnosis of a serious illness which would need treatment for some months.

"She said they (the girl's parents) both cried at the hospital," said my mother. She sampled my cakes, which were carefully made using wholemeal flour and honey instead of sugar but she did not like them and I watched, as she knelt on the kitchen floor, feeding pieces to the dog. She seemed entirely unaware that I was wondering how on earth *my* parents had been able to contemplate my own situation dispassionately!

A CHANGE

I began to be stronger and I felt refreshed, without the M.E. pallor — in fact, the opposite happened and I positively glowed! I could walk without difficulty and move freely; not only did I want to do my own chores, I was *able to do them!* I slept all night and was not desperate to nap during the daytime, although I was careful to rest for part of each afternoon. There really seemed to be more hours in each day than I could enjoy before this, for months.

Concentration improved and it was possible to read without getting sick and dizzy. In my car, I could raise my arms and hands to grasp the steering-wheel, move my legs to work the pedals — I began to drive again! When my older son's birthday came around I went out to choose his gifts and it felt great.

I went to a hairdresser and asked her to cut my hair into a sleek bob. As I began to put constant dishevelment behind me, I wore make-up and nail varnish, as I used to do. Reflections upon how many adverse comments there had been about my appearance over the previous two and a half years, as if I was somehow fair game, were depressing. Spiteful remarks included the information that I looked "older", "fed-up" and — always — "tired" .... ! (It is still a mystery to me, that my former, somewhat glamorous self was so readily forgotten by many friends and family members whilst I was ill! Was not the *state of me* a clue to my debilitation?)

BETTER!

I discovered a local M.E. support group and went to a meeting; at least, I meant to. However, although the couple who provided the venue were there, perhaps inevitably, no-one else came.

The woman who opened the door was friendly; she apologised for the absence of more visitors but seemed very keen for me to stay for a while and at first, took a real interest in my story. Her husband, an M.E. sufferer, made a brave attempt to join our discussion but he soon lost his strength and left the room to lie down. I saw the look on his face as energy deserted him and recognised it at once. When he tried again, after ten minutes, to come back to talk to me but failed, I was fascinated and saddened to witness a person enduring the misery I knew so well.

Together, the lady and I chatted for a little longer and I offered her some of the ideas I had developed but now she looked vague and told me she doubted diet would work; her husband ate as much as he could but in any case he had little appetite. In seconds and a few words, a valuable train of thought was dismissed! I was not yet well enough, myself, to put my case more forcibly, even if argument was appropriate. As I drove home, I reflected upon how obviously ill the poor man was. I *saw him* make a real effort to share conversation - he had to give up. In a confusion that has lasted ever since, I could not comprehend how my own suffering had been invisible.

Once I knew recovery was really happening, I had the long-awaited reward of being my "real self". The curious thing then, was the way people responded — accepting me, renewing acquaintance with my true character. Sadly I learned not to talk about my experience since it was never a welcome topic of conversation; I felt frustrated but there was nothing I could do. I must, at some point, have consciously decided not to challenge my family about it and that way forward became a habit. This may not have been quite the right plan since emotionally I felt whipped - yet I could not contemplate cutting anyone out of my life, although my marriage eventually ended at a later date.

Going on, I believed the key to staying well would be personal healthcare, coupled with an essential acute awareness of how emotional trauma can add to "overload". I had concerns about relapsing — feared it, really — but a few years later found I could enjoy riding horses again. I became well enough to notice occasionally, with hindsight, that for periods of time I actually took wellbeing for granted!

The removal of some foods from my diet during illness was not needed once I felt strong; it was not the same as (for instance) a dangerous peanut allergy. I can include some wine, a little chocolate and tea or coffee; however I still begin the day with camomile tea for its calming effect. Occasionally, I spot certain warning signs of a relapse, such as dizziness and I am quick to consider making dietary changes if I might be becoming unwell.

So: I was not actually ill **because of** my food but following a highly nutritious plan created a recovery. As for being active, if resting feels more important than exercising, I will rest, for it is impossible to forget my suffering and in fact I would be foolish to dismiss all the memories. However, the long nightmare of M.E. is over for me.

My Theories

The Collapsed Puppet

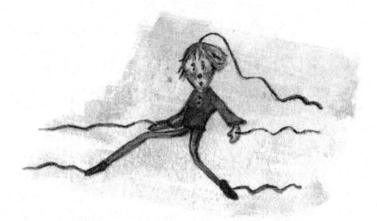

As a mother, any scrap of energy I had was for the care of my children. There were times when I would lie on the bed and feel I could not move, even to go to the bathroom. Some days I avoided the struggle to raise my arms to clean my teeth or — still harder — brush or wash my hair. If I was too hot, I could not change it — too cold, I shivered. No-one considered offering me personal care, so I had to wait. However, with recovery in mind, there were a few things I slowly began to change.

I thought of myself as a collapsed puppet. Weak and floppy, I imagined strings attached to my head, arms, hands and feet ... some strings thin, others thick and strong. I had to pull myself up very gently, getting hold of one fine strand of hope, at a time.

I stopped postponing a trip to the loo, even if I crept on all fours. (This will seem foolish to anyone who has not had or witnessed the same illness but I stand by my belief that one is truly clutching at straws; even fractional relief matters.) I cleaned my teeth, even if I spent just a few seconds on it and I dressed carefully for warmth or to be cool. No matter how I looked for the time being and if I was cold, I wrapped my head and neck in a scarf and abandoned any care about possible comment. Another good idea was to soak in a bath full of warm water, bringing myself back to a bearable temperature. On a nice day, I sat myself in the sunshine, deliberately raising my face for comfort and vitamin D.

To protect my emotions, I stopped paying attention to television news since I was unable to learn of harsh events without taking on board the suffering of others and if someone made a cruel comment, I recorded it in my diary (to get the feelings "spat out") then set it aside. I rested as much as I could. Above all, I slowly pulled the mighty string that was my diet.

The Beautiful Racehorse

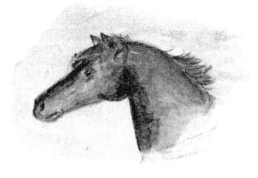

Bear with me if you know all about horses, it still works. For this fantasy, we pretend you are well or have a helper to order about and I am assuming a bossy style for once!

Imagine ... someone gives you an immaculate racehorse. No, you cannot say you don't want him, you have to have him, for a while! In the same way you cannot ignore your M.E., you *must* own the horse.

Needs: The horse is young, strong, glossy and on tiptoe with good health and fitness. In charge, you must keep him in this condition. Are you planning to do it with a tiny bit of unsuitable food, a splash of water, no bedding on the stone floor of the stable? Obviously not! If you know nothing about stable management, you need to find out what to do. Are you already a horse-lover? Aim to get things perfect.

Research: Find out how to address those needs, not just to keep the horse alive but also to make him fit for the races. You discover that clean water must always be available. As well as hay, feed and straw for the stable, the horse needs to be kept groomed and perhaps rugged-up. He will be unhappy if he is bored or lonely.

In the same way the horse can be cared-for to bring about the best chance of fitness, you can do that for yourself. A horse is not a person? Both are made of flesh & blood.

"He is well and I am ill?" It is about matching needs. A beautiful animal needs the right care, the optimum chance of survival AND fitness. You are not going to let him die, are you? (Please don't!) Wouldn't you, the new stable-hand, aim to do all the right things for the animal? I wanted to do this for myself, especially considering mine was not a task of maintenance but in an ill condition, to give myself the most chances I could find to become a well human being. Of course, the fantasy horse needs exercise (however, one would not ride him to the point of collapse) whilst an M.E. sufferer in recovery must rest, for now.

Welcome?

I was invited to a lunchtime gathering on a summer day and I was well enough to go! Everyone there knew I refused similar invitations for months. I could not share a Christmas dinner at my parents' house or keep in touch on the telephone for such a long time but at last there I was, leaning on a stick, smiling with relief. I trusted them to (at least) say: "Oh good, you must be feeling better!"

The reader may be forgiven for wondering how it was possible that I still looked for empathy! I knew there would be *no medal* but I assumed it was understood I had been through an awful experience. I had been hurt but I felt hopeful and after all, I had done nothing wrong.

Sadly, I had not fully comprehended that I no longer seemed to deserve respect. There must have been a shared perception that I actually *chose* to avoid socialising for all those months and contrary to my slender expectations, nobody said a single thing about my condition! There were glances at my stick but not at my face, as I stood uncertainly, feeling unreal. I had been lonely and it was exciting to prepare to go out yet now, I felt odd and out-of-place because, similarly to the way people sometimes behave after a bereavement, no-one seemed to know the right thing to say, so they pretended it did not happen.

As life went on I was never praised; my achievement was not acknowledged and even the kind aunt who sent the books thought it highly unlikely that I cured myself. Perhaps, subconsciously, I have been living with a sense of something missing! However, the story has been waiting to be told for twenty-six years and my favourite outcome would be if it helps someone, simply, to feel positive about a diagnosis of M.E.

POSTSCRIPT

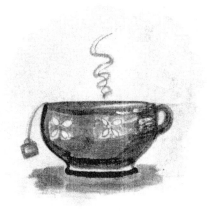

I have offered you this true story, in which I describe my experience of illness and recovery. Confusion about M.E. itself, coupled with disappointment in the responses of other people, had to be a part of it and who would not feel like a victim in the same situation? Determination followed and emotional reactions led eventually to a new mind-set and the discovery of a strength of character I never knew I possessed.

Sadly, I came out of all this thinking my life must be about heroics — lonely heroics, at that. It is no bad thing to understand that happy times are not one's automatic right and there are situations in which we must fight for the best outcome but if I could go back and whisper in my own ear, I would tell that younger "me" to remember *she deserved happiness*.

Review Requested:
If you loved this book, would you please provide a review at
Amazon.com?

CPSIA information can be obtained at www.ICGtesting.com
Printed in the USA
BVOW08*1003201016

465565BV00002B/5/P